PALEO COOKBOOK FOR ATHLETES

Lose Weight and Get Muscle Quickly and Easily

With the Paleo Solution

By Marc Holden

www.livingthefitness.com

amazon.com/author/marcholden

TABLE OF CONTENTS

50 PALEO RECIPES

Chicken Skewers with Broccoli	48
Chicken Livers with Scallions & Thyme	50
Lamb Stew with Pomegranates & Walnuts	52
Salmon in Parcel	54
Roasted Chicken with Root Vegetables	56
Baked Beef Stew	58
Roasted Beef Fore Rib	60
Roasted Lamb Leg with Mint Sauce	62
Roasted Chicken with Sweet Potatoes	64
Stir Fried Beef & Broccoli	66
Roasted Chicken with Creamy Butternut Squash	68
Chicken with Coconut Milk	70
Mushrooms Stuffed Roasted Chicken	72
Bacon with Apple & Avocado Salad	74
Crispy Chicken with Avocado	76
Butter & Herbs Stuffed Chicken	78
Stuffed Lamb Leg with Olives	80

INTRODUCTION

My name is Marc Holden, and I am an expert in fitness and well-being. With **YEARS** of experience behind me, you will find all the information you need in here to understand the power of the Paleo diet, but also how it can benefit you specifically.

Many people are built for different diets, and many of us do not have the discipline to go on some of the more extreme diets – this is the way of life. For those of us who are looking to get into the best shape you possibly can, then a Paleo diet is a pretty solid place to start.

It provides you with access to a wide variety of foods you will enjoy and regularly eat anyway, but the purpose of the diet is to keep the things you currently eat that benefit your system, but remove all of the negative products that are entering your system.

Although most of us probably eat too much fast food and enjoy the processed goods a little bit too much, a Paleo diet is not going to come as a huge shock to you. You still eat lots of very nice foods and you don't need to go cold turkey on enjoyable snacks, you simply replace them with an equally as tasty but more nutritious equivalent!

If you are ready to learn more about how to get your body in the best condition it can be, then keep reading – you are about to find some of the most interesting Paleo diet facts and help, which will make the entire process much easier to integrate in your life!

WHY THE PALEO DIET?

When starting any diet there should be two main questions you ask yourself, and they are:

- Why am I starting this diet?
- Can I live the life I need to with this diet?

If you cannot answer both of these questions in relation to any diet, then you need to get yourself something more suitable to your standards and style. So, what would the answers be if you were to start a Paleo diet?

To start off, the Paleo diet has been in circulation for about...two million years! About ten thousand years ago the human race changed its diet quite drastically when we started to eat things like grains and dairy. This is why so many people have intolerances to dairy, as our digestive system is not quite ready for it yet.

However, it has had a long, long time to get used to what you eat on a Paleo diet, which is the traditional stuff – fruits, vegetables, meats, nuts, and seeds. We have eaten this food for years and it has always been agreeable with our digestive systems, making it a no-brainer.

We have been eating the foods in a Paleo diet since day one, but with more modern foods like dairy, we have been consuming them for roughly 0.4% of our existence. Since we have moved into this new period of eating the foods we consume today, humanity has suffered quite a bit more with regards to health issues.

We have replaced the foods we use to eat with a series of low nutrition and high toxic meals that just damage our system, and do not provide it with what we need to live. Humanity has become smaller, we have more bone troubles these days, illnesses like cancer have become more common, diabetes is rife in certain countries, and things like skin problems and heart disease are on the rise constantly.

This is to do with our diets – before we changed to our current diets, we ate what made us healthy and made us strong. Today, we eat sugary goods that ruin our bodies over time and do untold damage.

A Paleo diet takes you back to your roots – it puts you back on a healthy lifestyle and removes all of the nonsense that we aren't ready to eat. Maybe in another 50,000 years our digestive system will be ready to cope with all of this junk, but today it is simply not prepared.

A Paleo diet cuts out all of the toxins we put into our systems and replaces them with natural supplements and nutrients, giving you a much healthier body as a result. Not only that, you are still given a huge amounts of foods to choose from when it comes to eating! So this is a fun diet to be on where you can mix it up and still enjoy your foods, all the while receiving the benefits you get from eating much cleaner!

CHARACTERICS OF A PALEO DIET

As we mentioned above, the Paleo diet still takes on many foods that we commonly eat today – berries, meats and fruits are all things we commonly pick up at the supermarket, especially meat. The Paleo diet is based on the foods that our ancestors would have eaten, back when we all gathered our own food and lived in small communities.

The Paleo diet is designed to take us back to that era, but it is also created to improve your health. Somebody who spends time on a Paleo diet will tend to notice the following changes to their system:

Better Protein Intake – In the average Western person's diet, protein makes up 15% of the calories we take in, which is around half of what our ancestors took in. Adding all of these foods rich in protein will improve your physical condition immeasurably.

Lower Glycemic Index – Glycemic is another term that is thrown about by dieticians, which is quite frightening sounding, but it actually has an important bearing on our system. On a Paleo diet, you make up roughly 45% of your foods with fresh fruits and vegetables without starch. This keeps your blood sugar levels nice and calm and you absorb the nutrients of the diet over time.

Source *Wikipedia*: *The glycemic index, or glycaemic index, (GI) provides a measure of how quickly blood sugar levels (i.e., levels of glucose in the blood) rise after eating a particular type of food. The effects that different foods have on blood sugar levels vary considerably. The glycemic index estimates how much each gram of available carbohydrate (total carbohydrate minus fiber) in a food raises a person's blood glucose level following consumption of the food, relative to consumption of pure glucose. Glucose has a glycemic index of 100.*

Better vitamin mix – Most of us get our vitamins through the little tablets or the chewy sweets, but we should be taking in much more vitamins in our body. The majority of the Western world suffers from a vitamin deficiency of some capacity, whereas in countries like India the vitamin deficiency level is much lower. Using a Paleo diet, you can restore your vitamin balance and leave yourself in rude health.

Balance your dietary acid – When we digest our food, it adds either alkaline or acid to our kidneys. Although meat and fish provide acid to our kidneys, fruits and vegetables offer an alkaline balance and with a Paleo diet you will find yourself much more balanced, cancelling each other out. This cuts down on the chances of things like asthma and kidney stones.

More potassium, less sodium – Foods, which aren't processed contain roughly ten times more potassium than sodium. Potassium helps your organs work properly, and gets your heart and kidneys in order – without the extra potassium, your chances of heart attacks and blood pressure problems are much higher.

As you can see, the Paleo diet puts you in the position where you can provide a much more powerful balance to your diet, allowing you to enjoy a much more comfortable life. By removing these potential health risks and improving your general condition, you will find that the Paleo diet offers many methods to cut your health problems down and give you a much more balanced diet for the future.

GETTING STARTED WITH PALEO

As you can tell now, the Paleo diet is not designed just to get you in better shape – it is far more than that. It puts you in a real athletes mindset as you move away from eating the less damaging foods and get yourself toward a much more complete and comfortable lifestyle.

Getting started is fairly easy – based on eating wholesome foods, which provide health benefits rather than just fill you up until the next meal, the Paleo diet is easy to start as you have all of the foods available in supermarkets and markets.

You need to start off by clearing out all of the foods in your house that are no longer suitable for a Paleo diet – by removing temptation you will find it much easier to stick to the diet and see the true benefits.

Next, make sure your shopping list is now modified to pick up a variety of foods that suit a Paleo diet. Read on to find the right information about what you can and cannot eat. Having been researched for years, the Paleo diet is a certainty to help you get into much better shape – not only can it help combat years of lazy eating but the choices are enjoyable and easy to mix into different meals keeping the diet fresh and interesting.

Struggling for motivation? Look online and check out the chances of contracting the following illnesses in your country:

- Cancer
- Diabetes
- Myopia
- Acne
- Osteoporosis
- Sclerosis
- IBS
- Crohn's Disease
- Gout
- Varicose veins
- Hemorrhoids
- Gastric reflux
- Heart problems

Now, not all of these are life threatening but some of them are extremely serious! However, by moving your diet towards a Paleo diet you can significantly reduce your chances of contracting any of the above. If that isn't motivation for you, I don't know what would be!

WHAT & WHAT NOT TO EAT

The Paleo diet is one of those enjoyable diets, as it takes you into a much more open-minded theme when it comes to food consumption. Many diets rule out just about anything we enjoy, making it hard to stick to your diet. But when you get a diet like this that provides you with healthy eating that is good for you as well as enjoyable, then you know you have found a winner.

Although the list can break down a lot deeper than this – you can be fairly safe in the knowledge that any food, which falls under the 'What' category is safe, and what falls under the 'What Not' category, is something you should avoid at all costs;

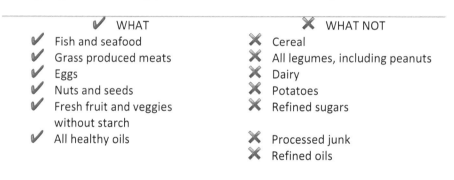

✔ WHAT	✖ WHAT NOT
✔ Fish and seafood	✖ Cereal
✔ Grass produced meats	✖ All legumes, including peanuts
✔ Eggs	✖ Dairy
✔ Nuts and seeds	✖ Potatoes
✔ Fresh fruit and veggies without starch	✖ Refined sugars
✔ All healthy oils	✖ Processed junk
	✖ Refined oils

Some of us struggle to adapt to this list above, as it cuts out things we eat out of habit and such, or we don't see instant results and instantly disregard it. Don't worry though, even athletes can struggle to get to grips with the Paleo diet, it is certainly tough to get into it but when you do – you should have no problems sustaining it!

Some people think that to do a Paleo diet you need to actually go out with the sword and the rifle and hunt down some food for yourself – this is not the suggestion at all! You can live your life exactly as it is, you just cut out all of the madness and junk that you take in.

Although you may be giving up things like bread or toast and favorites like spaghetti, you need to open your mind and remind yourself that with the Paleo diet you will be trying lots of very different foods and products, which make adjusting a little bit easier. Most diets restrict you to a finite amount, making it harder to adapt and stick to it. However, with a Paleo diet you should have no such worries.

CREATING YOUR OWN FOOD PLANS

In due time, you will want to come up with your own ideas for food plans and you will like to keep the diet fresh and exciting. The main problem most people have with diets is running out of selections and beginning a really monotonous food structure where your weekdays take in the exact same foods as the week before.

However, with the Paleo diet you don't have this problem. Because the options available to you are still pretty large and varied, you can really mix things up and make the most of your options out there.

For many people, the target aim is roughly 80-20. This means you eat well and healthy 80% of the time, and eat how you please the other 20%. Of course, the balance you want is 100-0, but if you cannot attain that then 80-20 is a good starting point.

The Paleo diet is all about commitments and sticking to it, and it is much easier to do if you can create your own food plans. I provide you in this book with a series of recipes, which you can start making today, but at the moment here is the general consensus about how you should go about creating your own Paleo menu:

UNDERSTAND THE WHAT AND WHAT NOT SECTION!

The section that precedes this, 'What' and 'What Not' to eat gives you all the information you might need about the Paleo diet and what you can put in. However, drilling down beyond the type of food is important too and ask yourself what you are actually buying.

Are you buying good, genuine meat or is it a processed piece of slurp? Are you getting the right type of oils for your foods? The only fats you should really be taking in are from oils. Getting your head around the list above will make shopping trips much less confusing – I mean, there are more than seven types of meats out there you can legitimately eat and enjoy with this diet, so if you have meat as your main dinner course every night – as you probably do most nights anyway – then you just need to substitute your sides like chips with something a little more healthy.

PREPARE YOURSELF

If you are going to get involved in the Paleo diet, then you need to realize how big of a factor it will be playing in your lifestyle. When you start the diet, you need to keep going as starting and stopping is pointless – this is why before you start, you should spend some time preparing yourself.

Prepare all of your food beforehand, have a meal list for the entire week decided on a Sunday that gives you the chance to try out different things and actually go out of the box a little bit, while remaining true to the diet itself.

Creating your own plans is all about finding new recipes to keep your food nice and simple, and we will give your over fifty different, totally unique, recipes for your own pleasure!

This means that preparing your house for the right type of food and setting yourself to live a much healthier life from this day forward is vital – without that preparation, it can be harder to stick to the plan.

Conclusion

I hope that within this book you have found the information helpful and insightful, and I really do hope that you are considering going for the Paleo diet. Reading through here, you must have about ten reasons why you should be changing for the long-term!

- It provides much better health benefits than other diets
- It provides MUCH better health benefits to sticking to your current diet!
- It creates a flexible and enjoyable menu, despite helping you lose weight and live better
- A common choice for athletes, this is a lifestyle choice as much as a diet. It takes time and patience but the long-term benefits are massive
- Cuts down on the risk of serious illnesses massively
- Live longer
- Create a sustained system where you will find that you have more energy and motivation to get things done
- Puts yourself in a position where you will be able to achieve more
- Disciplines yourself away from the modern junk that we all eat
- Gives your family a better lifestyle, not just yourself

By sticking to a Paleo diet, you can find that your lifestyle changes totally – you will feel more active, more prepared and energized. It not only benefits you to help you lose weight, but it puts you in a position where you can achieve more and really push forward with your life!

Are you ready to change, cut out the last 10,000 years of disgusting food, and put yourself on the track to a healthier body and better life? Then get started today!

I really hope this inspires you to start and to thoroughly enjoy your life from here on in – it is hard work, but when you get going you will not want to look back!

Thanks for your time, hope to see you enjoying your Paleo diet soon!

SCRAMBLED EGGS WITH CHICKEN & CHERRY TOMATOES

Prep Time: 10 minutes

Cooking Time: 5 minutes

Serves: 4

INGREDIENTS

8 large eggs

4 egg whites

Salt and black pepper, to taste

1 teaspoon dried thyme

3 tablespoons almond butter

1 cup cooked chicken, shredded

2 cups cherry tomatoes, halved

4 small jalapeño, seeded and chopped

4 scallions, chopped

PREPARATIONS

1. In a bowl, add eggs, egg whites, salt, black pepper, and thyme and whisk well.
2. In a large frying pan, heat butter over medium-low heat. Add chicken, tomatoes, and jalapeños and cook for 2 to 3 minutes.
3. Add egg mixture and cook, stirring for 4 to 5 minutes or till eggs are done completely.
4. Stir in scallions and cook for 1 to 2 minutes.

NUTRITION FACTS PER SERVING:

Calories: 307
Fat: 18.0g
Carbohydrates: 7.3g
Fiber: 1.8g
Sugar: 3.3g
Protein: 29.8g

Mini Meatloaves

Prep Time: 10 minutes

Cooking Time: 30 minutes

Serves: 4

Ingredients

2 tablespoons coconut oil

1 medium yellow onion

1 pound cooked beef, shredded finely

1 egg, beaten lightly

2 tablespoons fresh thyme leaves, chopped

1 tablespoon fresh sage leaves, chopped

¼ teaspoon ground all spices

¼ teaspoon ground nutmeg

2 teaspoons fennel seeds

Salt and black pepper, to taste

4 eggs, hard-boiled

Preparations

1. Preheat the oven to 325 degrees F.(170 degrees C) Lightly, grease a baking dish.
2. In a pan, heat oil on medium heat. Add onion and sauté till soft.
3. In a large bowl, add sautéed onion and remaining ingredients and mix till well combined.
4. Make 4 thin patties from meat mixture.
5. Place a boiled egg in the center. Fold the meat to cover the egg completely.
6. Place the mini meatloaves in prepared baking dish.
7. Bake for 20 to 25 minutes.

Nutrition Facts Per Serving:

Calories: 310
Fat: 12.9g
Carbohydrates: 4.7g
Fiber: 1.7g
Sugar: 1.6g
Protein: 41.9g

Chicken & Eggs Casserole

Prep Time: 10 minutes

Cooking Time: 1 hour 10 minutes

Serves: 4

Ingredients

1 tablespoon coconut oil

1 pound boneless chicken, cut into bite sized pieces

4 eggs, beaten

3 turnips, peeled and grated

4 scallions, chopped

Salt and black pepper, to taste

PREPARATIONS

1. Preheat the oven to 400 degrees F (200 degrees C). Lightly grease a casserole dish.
2. In a pan, heat oil on medium heat. Add chicken and sauté for 4 to 5 minutes or until browned.
3. In a large bowl, add all ingredients and mix well.
4. Place the chicken mixture in prepared casserole dish.
5. Cover and bake for 45 minutes.
6. Uncover and bake for 15 to 20 minutes more.

NUTRITION FACTS PER SERVING

Calories: 339

Fat: 16.2g

Carbohydrates: 7.5g

Fiber: 1.9g

Sugar: 4.4g

Protein: 39.4g

BEEF & TURNIP SCRAMBLE

Prep Time: 10 minutes

Cooking Time: 20 minutes

Serves: 4

INGREDIENTS

2 tablespoon coconut oil

1 pound boneless beef, cut into bite sized pieces

1 pound turnips, peeled and grated

Salt and black pepper, to taste

4 eggs, beaten

4 scallions, chopped

¼ cup fresh basil, chopped

1. In a skillet, heat oil on medium heat. Add beef and cook for 8 to 10 minutes.
2. Add grated turnips and season with salt and black pepper. Cook for 5 minutes.
3. Add eggs and cook for 4 to 5 minutes or till done completely.
4. Stir in scallions and basil and serve.

NUTRITION FACTS PER SERVING

Calories: 291
Fat: 11.6g
Carbohydrates: 8.0g
Fiber: 2.1g
Sugar: 4.8g
Protein: 37.0g

Scrambled Eggs with Lamb & Scallions

Prep Time: 10 minutes

Cooking Time: 1 minute

Serves: 4

Ingredients

1 medium butternut squash, peeled and shredded

½ cup scallions, sliced

1/3 pound cooked lamb, shredded

6 eggs

¼ cup flax meal

1/3 cup coconut milk

Salt and black pepper, to taste

PREPARATIONS

1. Preheat the oven to 350 degrees F (175 degrees C). Lightly grease a casserole dish.
2. Place butternut squash in the bottom of prepared casserole dish.
3. Spread scallions and shredded lamb over butternut squash.
4. In a blender, add remaining ingredients and blend until smooth.
5. Spread egg mixture over lamb evenly.
6. Bake for 45 minutes.

NUTRITION FACTS PER SERVING

Calories: 296
Fat: 18.0g
Carbohydrates: 8.6g
Fiber: 3.5g
Sugar: 2.2g
Protein: 26.8g

Eggs & Chicken Squares

Prep Time: 10 minutes

Cooking Time: 35 minutes

Serves: 4

Ingredients

2 tablespoons coconut butter

1 bunch fresh spinach

2 ½ cups cooked chicken, shredded

8 eggs

1 bunch parsley

Salt and black pepper, to taste

PREPARATIONS

1. Preheat the oven to 375 degrees F (175 degrees C). Lightly grease a baking dish.
2. In a pan, melt butter on medium heat.
3. Sauté spinach for 4 to 5 minutes.
4. Add chicken and cook for 3 to 4 minutes.
5. Beat eggs in a bowl. Add spinach, chicken, parsley, salt and black pepper and mix well.
6. Place egg mixture in prepared baking dish.
7. Bake for 20 to 25 minutes.
8. Let it cool slightly. Then cut into 4 squares.

NUTRITION FACTS PER SERVING

Calories: 394
Fat: 22.4g
Carbohydrates: 8.8g
Fiber: 5.4g
Sugar: 2.2g
Protein: 40.3g

POACHED EGGS WITH CHICKEN & TOMATOES

Prep Time: 10 minutes

Cooking Time: 30 minutes

Serves: 4

INGREDIENTS

¼ cup coconut oil

1 large white onion, chopped

1 green bell pepper, seeded and chopped

1 red bell pepper, seeded and chopped

1 cup cooked chicken, shredded finely

4 cloves garlic, chopped finely

½ teaspoon ground cumin

2 ½ pounds fresh tomatoes, chopped finely

8 eggs

Salt and black pepper, to taste

½ cup fresh parsley, chopped

PREPARATIONS

1. Preheat the oven to 400 degrees F (200 degrees C).
2. In an ovenproof skillet, heat oil on medium-high heat.
3. Add onion and bell peppers and chicken and sauté for 5 minutes.
4. Add garlic and cumin and cook for 1 minute.
5. Add tomatoes and reduce heat to medium-low. Simmer for 15 to 20 minutes or till most of the liquid is absorbed.
6. Season with salt and black pepper.
7. Crack the eggs in the skillet evenly.
8. Place the skillet in the preheated oven.
9. Bake for 6 to 8 minutes.
10. Garnish with parsley before serving.

NUTRITION FACTS PER SERVING

Calories: 389
Fat: 24.2g
Carbohydrates: 20.3g
Fiber: 5.8g
Sugar: 12.2g
Protein: 25.2g

Bacon & Kale Frittata

Prep Time: 10 minutes

Cooking Time: 40 minutes

Serves: 4

Ingredients

2 tablespoons coconut oil

1 pound bacon, cut into ½-inch bits

1 small red bell pepper, seeded and chopped

2 cups kale, trimmed and chopped

1 small onion, chopped

Salt and black pepper, to taste

8 eggs, beaten

1/3 cup coconut milk

1. Preheat the oven to 375 degrees F (180 degrees C). Lightly grease a baking dish.
2. In a non-stick pan, heat 1 tablespoon of oil on medium heat. Cook bacon for 4 to 5 minutes or till crisp. Transfer bacon from pan into a plate.
3. In the same pan, add bell pepper, kale, and onion and sauté for 3 to 4 minutes.
4. In a large bowl, mix together bacon and vegetables and season with salt and black pepper.
5. In a bowl, beat eggs. Ad coconut milk some salt and black pepper and mix well.
6. Place bacon mixture in the bottom of prepared basking dish.
7. Pour egg mixture over bacon mixture evenly.
8. Bake for 30 minutes.

NUTRITION FACTS PER SERVING

Calories: 818
Fat: 66.4g
Carbohydrates: 9.4g
Fiber: 2.4g
Sugar: 3.6g
Protein: 45.7g

Chicken & Mushrooms Muffins

Prep Time: 10 minutes

Cooking Time: 35 minutes

Serves: 4

Ingredients

4 tablespoons coconut oil

1 cup boneless chicken, cut into bite size pieces

1 small onion, chopped finely

½ pound cremini mushrooms, sliced thinly

½ pound fresh spinach, trimmed and chopped

8 large eggs

¼ cup coconut milk

2 tablespoons coconut flour

1 cup cherry tomatoes, halved

Salt and black pepper to taste

PREPARATIONS

1. Preheat the oven to 375 degrees F (180 degrees C). Lightly grease a 12 muffin cup tray.
2. In a skillet, heat oil on medium heat.
3. Add chicken and cook for 5 minutes. Remove chicken from pan.
4. Add onion and sauté for 4 to 5 minutes.
5. Add mushrooms and garlic and cook for 4 to 5 minutes. Season with salt and black pepper.
6. Add spinach and cook for 2 to 3 minutes.
7. In a large bowl add eggs, coconut milk, coconut flour, salt and black pepper and whisk till well mixed. Add in chicken, mushrooms and spinach and mix well.
8. Place the egg mixture in muffin cups evenly. Top with halved cherry tomatoes.
9. Bake for 20 minutes.

NUTRITION FACTS PER SERVING

Calories: 423
Fat: 19.3g
Carbohydrates: 11.0g
Fiber: 4.0g
Sugar: 4.4g
Protein: 27.3g

Chicken, Sweet Potatoes & Zucchini Frittata

Prep Time: 10 minutes

Cooking Time: 25 minutes

Serves: 4

Ingredients

3 tablespoons coconut butter

1/3 pound chicken, cut into bite size pieces

1 small sweet potato, peeled and cubed

1 zucchinis, pealed and sliced

1 small red bell pepper, seeded and sliced

8 large eggs

2 tablespoon parsley, chopped

Salt and black pepper, to taste

PREPARATIONS

1. In a pan, melt butter on medium heat.
2. Add chicken and cook for 4 to 5 minutes. Transfer chicken in to a plate.
3. In the same pan, add sweet potatoes. Cook for 8 o 10 minutes on medium-low heat.
4. Add zucchini and bell pepper and cook for 4 to 5 minutes.
5. In a bowl, whisk eggs with parsley, salt and black pepper.
6. Return chicken into pan and pour egg mixture in.
7. Reduce heat to low. Cook for 10 minutes.

NUTRITION FACTS PER SERVING

Calories: 254
Fat: 7.8g
Carbohydrates: 8.8g
Fiber: 1.9g
Sugar: 3.6g
Protein: 35.8g

Beef & Beans Salad

Prep Time: 10 minutes

Cooking Time: 10 minutes

Serves: 4

Ingredients

½ pounds fresh beans, trimmed

Salt and black pepper, to taste

1 pound boneless beef fillet, sliced thinly

2 sprigs of fresh thyme

2 tablespoons coconut oil

For Salad

1 red onion

2 tablespoons fresh parsley, chopped

1½ teaspoon Dijon mustard

2 tablespoons fresh lime juice

4 tablespoons extra virgin olive oil

1. In a pan of boiling water, add beans and cook for 5 minutes. Drain and keep aside.
2. In a bowl, add beef, salt, black pepper, and thyme and mix well.
3. In a pan, heat oil on medium heat.
4. Add beef and stir-fry for 4 to 5 minutes.
5. In a large bowl, add all salad ingredients and toss to coat well.
6. Serve beef slices with salad.

NUTRITION FACTS PER SERVING

Calories: 314
Fat: 14.1g
Carbohydrates: 11.0g
Fiber: 4.5g
Sugar: 2.8g
Protein: 36.8g

Grilled Steak with Spinach Salad

Prep Time: 10 minutes

Cooking Time: 10 minutes

Serves: 4

Ingredients

For Salad

1½ pounds grilled beefsteak, cut into thin strips

8 cups baby spinach

1 large red onion, sliced thinly

¼ cup pecans

¼ cup walnuts

For Dressing

1/3 cup olive oil

3 tablespoons

½ cup fresh lemon juice

2 teaspoons garlic, minced finely

Salt and black pepper, to taste

PREPARATIONS

1. In a bowl, add all salad ingredients and mix well.
2. In another bowl, add all dressing ingredients and whisk till well combined.
3. Pour Dressing over salad. Toss to coat well.

NUTRITION FACTS PER SERVING

Calories: 298
Fat: 15.3g
Carbohydrates: 34.6g
Fiber: 5.5g
Sugar: 13.4g
Protein: 19.6g

Salmon, Apple & Spinach Salad

Prep Time: 15 minutes

Cooking Time: 10 minutes

Serves: 4

Ingredients

For Salad

1½ pounds salmon fillets

8 cups baby spinach

6 cups lettuce

2 cups cabbage, shredded

1 green apple, cored and sliced thinly

For Dressing

1 cup walnut oil

2 tablespoons apple cider vinegar

1 large shallot, minced

Salt and black pepper, to taste

1. Preheat the oven o 350 degrees F (175 degrees C).
2. Place salmon fillets in a baking dish. Season with salt and pepper.
3. Add some water to gust cover fish. Cover with a foil paper. Bake for 10 minutes.
4. In a large bowl, add salad ingredients and mix.
5. In another bowl, add all dressing ingredients and whisk till well combined.
6. Pour dressing over salad and toss to coat.
7. Serve salad with fish fillets.

NUTRITION FACTS PER SERVING

Calories: 605
Fat: 39.8g
Carbohydrates: 16.5g
Fiber: 6.4g
Sugar: 8.1g
Protein: 48.1g

Grilled Chops with Herbs

Prep Time: 10 minutes

Cooking Time: 6 hours 10 minutes

Serves: 4

Ingredients

3 tablespoons coconut oil

2 cloves garlic, minced

¼ cup fresh parsley, chopped

¼ cup fresh thyme, chopped

Zest of 1 lemon, grated

Salt and black pepper, to taste

1 ½ pounds lamb chops

1. In a bowl, add all ingredients and mix till well coated.
2. Cover and refrigerate for 4 to 6 hours to marinate.
3. Remove chops from refrigerator 1 hour before grilling.
4. Preheat the grill to medium heat.
5. Grill chops 3 to 4 minutes per side.

NUTRITION FACTS PER SERVING

Calories: 420
Fat: 23.0g
Carbohydrates: 4.0g
Fiber: 1.7g
Sugar: 0.0g
Protein: 48.4g

Chicken Skewers with Broccoli

Prep Time: 25 minutes

Cooking Time: 15 minutes

Serves: 4

Ingredients

5 tablespoons coconut oil, melted and divided

2 tablespoons dried marjoram

2 cloves garlic, minced

2 tablespoons tomato paste (home made)

Salt and black pepper, to taste

16 boneless chicken tenderloin

4 cups broccoli, cut into florets

2 teaspoons extra-virgin olive oil

Preparations

1. In a bowl, add 4 tablespoons oil, marjoram, garlic, tomato paste, salt and black pepper and mix well.
2. Add chicken and coat well.
3. Keep aside for 10 to 15 minutes.
4. Thread chicken in pre-soaked skewers.
5. In large frying pan, heat remaining coconut oil. Add chicken skewers and cook for 4 to 5 minutes per side.
6. Meanwhile cook broccoli in boiling water for 3 to 4 minutes.
7. Toss broccoli with olive oil. Season with salt and black pepper.
8. Serve chicken with broccoli.

Nutrition Facts per Serving

Calories: 578
Fat: 18.4g
Carbohydrates: 8.4g
Fiber: 3.0g
Sugar: 2.5g
Protein: 91.0g

Chicken Livers with Scallions & Thyme

Prep Time: 10 minutes

Cooking Time: 15 minutes

Serves: 4

Ingredients

1½ pounds chicken livers, halved

Salt and black pepper, to taste

2 tablespoons coconut oil

2 scallions, sliced

1 tablespoon fresh lemon juice

2 tablespoons coconut butter

3 cloves garlic, chopped

10 sprigs of thyme, tied with a kitchen string

Preparations

1. In a bowl, add chicken livers. Sprinkle with a little salt and black pepper.
2. In a pan, heat oil and sauté scallions for 4 to 5 minutes.
3. Drizzle lemon juice and keep aside.
4. In another pan, heat butter on medium-high heat. Add garlic and sprigs of thyme and cook for 2 to 3 minutes. Transfer garlic and thyme sprigs to a plate.
5. Add chicken livers in the same pan and cook for 4 to 5 minutes, turning once.
6. Stir in sautéed scallions, garlic, and thyme and season with salt and black pepper.
7. Remove from heat and serve.

Nutrition Facts per Serving

Calories: 482
Fat: 29.1g
Carbohydrates: 11.7g
Fiber: 6.1g
Sugar: 1.4g
Protein: 43.6g

Lamb Stew with Pomegranates & Walnuts

Prep Time: 10 minutes

Cooking Time: 1 hour 45 minutes

Serves: 4

INGREDIENTS

1½ pounds roasting lamb, cubed

2 tablespoons almond flour

Salt and black pepper, to taste

2 tablespoons coconut oil

1 red onion, sliced finely

4 cloves garlic, sliced finely

4 sticks celery, trimmed and sliced finely

2 bay leaves

1 small stick cinnamon

½ cup walnuts, chopped

2 cups fresh pomegranate juice

1 bunch fresh parsley, chopped

1. In a bowl, add cubed lamb, flour, salt and black pepper and toss to coat.
2. In a large skillet, heat oil on medium heat. Add lamb and cook for 8 to 10 minutes or till soft and brown.
3. Add remaining ingredients except pomegranate juice and parsley. Cook, stirring often for 5 minutes.
4. Pour pomegranate juice and some water to cover the lamb.
5. Reduce heat to medium-low. Simmer for 1½ hours.
6. Remove from heat and discard bay leaves and cinnamon stick.
7. Garnish with parsley and serve.

NUTRITION FACTS PER SERVING

Calories: 676
Fat: 37.0g
Carbohydrates: 31.2g
Fiber: 3.9g
Sugar: 18.7g
Protein: 56.0g

Salmon in Parcel

Prep Time: 1 day 10 minutes

Cooking Time: 30 minutes

Serves: 4

Ingredients

2 eggs

2 cups sweet potatoes, cubed

1¼ pounds salmon fillets, skinned

2 lemons, sliced

2 bulbs fennel, trimmed and cut into wedges

20 cherry tomatoes

1 cup black olives, pitted

1 teaspoon olive oil

Salt and black pepper, to taste

PREPARATIONS

1. Make bags with foil paper by folding it double. Fold three sides and seal with beaten egg. Keep aside.
2. Add potatoes in boiling water and cook for 4 to 5 minutes.
3. Meanwhile in a bowl, add remaining ingredients and mix well.
4. Drain the potatoes and mix with other ingredients.
5. Place the fish mixture in prepared bags. Seal the remaining edges of the parcels. Refrigerate the parcels for a whole day.
6. Preheat the oven to 400 degrees F (200 degrees C). Line a baking dish.
7. Reseal the parcel bag and place them over prepared baking dish.
8. Bake for 20 to 25 minutes.

NUTRITION FACTS PER SERVING

Calories: 629
Fat: 29.1g
Carbohydrates: 47.2g
Fiber: 11.7g
Sugar: 16.5g
Protein: 47.3g

ROASTED CHICKEN WITH ROOT VEGETABLES

Prep Time: 10 minutes

Cooking Time: 1 minute

Serves: 4

INGREDIENTS

½ cup almond butter, softened

Zest of 2 lemons

1 bunch fresh thyme, divided

Salt and black pepper, to taste

2 pounds whole chicken

2 tablespoons plus 1 tablespoon coconut oil

1 lemon, sliced

1 bulb, garlic, sliced

1 pound mixed root vegetables (parsnips, carrots and sweet potatoes)

PREPARATIONS

1. Preheat the oven to 400 degrees F (200 degrees C).
2. In a bowl, mix together butter, lemon zest, and leaves from half of thyme sprig, salt and black pepper.
3. Place the chicken in roasting pan. Rub with the butter mixture generously. Drizzle oil over chicken evenly.
4. Stuff lemon slices and remaining thyme sprig inside the chicken cavity.
5. Roast chicken for 1 hour and 15 minutes.
6. Meanwhile in a pan of boiling water, add parsnips and carrots and cook for 5 to 6 minutes.
7. Add sweet potatoes and cook for 4 minutes more.
8. Drain vegetables and let them cool.
9. Place vegetables on a baking sheet. Drizzle with remaining oil and season with salt and black pepper.
10. Just 45 minutes before chicken is done, place the baking sheet with vegetables in oven.

NUTRITION FACTS PER SERVING

Calories: 771
Fat: 45.1g
Carbohydrates: 17.7g
Fiber: 6.7g
Sugar: 1.1g
Protein: 74.3g

Baked Beef Stew

Prep Time: 10 minutes

Cooking Time: 4 hours 5 minutes

Serves: 4

Ingredients

1 tablespoon coconut butter

3 tablespoons almond butter

1 pound stew beef meat, cubed

2 tablespoons almond flour

Salt and black pepper

1 medium onion, chopped

2 tablespoons fresh sage, chopped

4 carrots, peeled and chopped

2 parsnips, peeled and quartered

½ butternut squash, seeded and diced

½ pound sweet potatoes, peeled and diced

2 tablespoons artichokes, peeled and halved

3 tablespoons, tomato puree (home made)

1½ cup beef broth

Zest of 1 lemon, grated

2 tablespoons fresh rosemary, chopped

PREPARATIONS

1. Preheat the oven to 300 degrees F (150 degrees C). Lightly grease a baking dish.
2. In a bowl, add meat, flour, salt and black pepper and toss to coat. Keep aside.
3. In a pan, heat butter on medium heat. Add onion and sage and sauté for 3 minutes.
4. Add meat and vegetables, tomato puree, and beef broth in the pan
5. Season with salt and black pepper. Bring to a boil and cook for 2 minutes.
6. Transfer the mixture in prepared baking dish.
7. Cover and bake for 3 to 4 hours or beef is done completely.

NUTRITION FACTS PER SERVING

Calories: 524
Fat: 24.3g
Carbohydrates: 33.6g
Fiber: 8.1g
Sugar: 6.2g
Protein: 44.2g

Roasted Beef Fore Rib

Prep Time: 10 minutes

Cooking Time: 1 minute

Serves: 4

Ingredients

1 pound fresh beetroots, peeled and halved

4 cloves garlic, minced and divided

2 tablespoons fresh rosemary, chopped

Zest of 1 lemon, grated

Salt and black pepper, to taste

2 tablespoons coconut oil

2 pounds beef fore rib, trimmed and tied

¼ cup fresh lemon juice, divided

1 tablespoon fresh parsley, chopped

½ cup coconut cream

1 tablespoon fresh horse radish, peeled and grated

1. Preheat the oven to 400 degrees F (200 degrees C).
2. Add beetroots in salted water filled pan and bring to a boil. Reduce the heat. Simmer for 50 minutes.
3. In a large bowl, mix together 2 cloves garlic, rosemary, lemon zest, salt, black pepper, and 1½ tablespoons of oil. Rub the marinade over beef generously.
4. Place beef rib in a roasting tray. Roast for 1 hour.
5. Drain beetroots well. Place them in a bowl.
6. In the same bowl, add remaining garlic, 2 tablespoons of lemon juice, thyme, and remaining oil and toss well.
7. After 1 hour remove roasting tray from oven.
8. Spread the beetroots around beef in the tray.
9. Place the tray again in the oven. Roast for 30 minutes more.
10. In a bowl, add remaining lemon juice, parsley, cream, and horseradish. Season with salt and pepper and mix well.
11. Serve roasted beef and beetroots with flavored cream.

NUTRITION FACTS PER SERVING

Calories: 430
Fat: 28.7g
Carbohydrates: 16.7g
Fiber: 4.2g
Sugar: 12.3g
Protein: 27.7g

Roasted Lamb Leg with Mint Sauce

Prep Time: 10 minutes

Cooking Time: 1 hour 10 minutes

Serves: 4

Ingredients

For Roasted Leg

1 pound sweet potatoes, peeled and cubed

4 tablespoons coconut oil

8 cloves garlic, crushed and divided

Zest of 1 lemon

1 bunch of fresh rosemary, divided

1 pound lamb leg

Salt and black pepper, to taste

1 pound sweet potatoes, peeled and cubed

For Mint Sauce

2 tablespoons fresh mint leaves, chopped

12 tablespoons hot water

1 tablespoon fresh lemon juice

½ teaspoon coconut sugar

Pinch of salt

PREPARATIONS

1. Preheat the oven to 400 degrees F/200 degrees C.
2. Add sweet potatoes in water filled pan and cook for 10 minutes. Drain them.
3. In a bowl, add sweet potatoes, 2 tablespoons of oil and 3 cloves of garlic. Season with salt and black pepper. Toss to coat.
4. In a large bowl, mix together 2 tablespoons of oil, 5 cloves garlic, lemon zest, and chopped rosemary leaves of half sprig. Rub the marinade over lamb generously. Season with salt and black pepper.
5. Place lamb leg on the hot bars of the oven above the tray.
6. Spread sweet potatoes in roasting tray and place under the lamb.
7. Roast the lamb for 1 hour.
8. Meanwhile in a bowl, mix together all sauce ingredients.
9. Serve roasted lamb with sweet potatoes and mint sauce.

NUTRITION FACTS PER SERVING
Calories: 703
Fat: 39.2g
Carbohydrates: 67.4g
Fiber: 10.1g
Sugar: 2.1g
Protein: 23.2g

Roasted Chicken with Sweet Potatoes

Prep Time: 12 hours

Cooking Time: 1 hour 40 minutes

Serves: 4

Ingredients

2 pounds whole chicken

Salt and black pepper, to taste

1 pound sweet potatoes, peeled and cubed

5 cloves garlic

1 large lemon, wedged

2 tablespoons fresh thyme, chopped

2 tablespoons fresh rosemary, chopped

3 tablespoons coconut oil

1. With a sharp knife, make deep cuts in chicken.
2. Rub salt and black pepper generously.
3. Refrigerate for 10 to 12 hours to marinate.
4. Preheat the oven to 375 degrees F (180 degrees C).
5. In a pan of boiling water, add sweet potatoes, garlic and lemon. Cook for 8 to 10 minutes.
6. Drain sweet potatoes.
7. Place hot lemon, garlic cloves, and thyme in the cavity of the chicken.
8. Drizzle oil on chicken generously.
9. Place chicken in roasting pan and roast for 45 minutes.
10. After 45 minutes place sweet potatoes around chicken.
11. Roast for 45 minutes more.

Nutrition Facts per Serving

Calories: 384
Fat: 12.2g
Carbohydrates: 32.9g
Fiber: 5.3g
Sugar: 0.6g
Protein: 34.7g

Stir Fried Beef & Broccoli

Prep Time: 10 minutes

Cooking Time: 15 minutes

Serves: 4

Ingredients

¼ pound broccoli, sliced

Salt and black pepper, to taste

1 pound beef steaks, sliced thinly

3 teaspoons ground coriander

3 tablespoons coconut oil

1 medium onion, sliced finely

1 (1-inch) piece fresh ginger, chopped finely

3 cloves garlic, sliced

1. Add broccoli in a bowl of boiling water. Add some salt and keep aside for 10 minutes.
2. Season beef with salt, black pepper, and coriander.
3. In a skillet, heat oil on medium heat.
4. Add onion, ginger and garlic and sauté for 4 to 5 minutes.
5. Add beef and stir-fry for 6 to 8 minutes.
6. Add drained broccoli and stir-fry for 2 minutes more.

NUTRITION FACTS PER SERVING

Calories: 291

Fat: 10.9g

Carbohydrates: 10.3g

Fiber: 3.5g

Sugar: 3.0g

Protein: 37.9g

Roasted Chicken with Creamy Butternut Squash

Prep Time: 10 minutes

Cooking Time: 35 minutes

Serves: 4

Ingredients

4 (4-ounce each) chicken breasts

2 fresh red chilies, seeded and sliced

5 sprigs fresh oregano, chopped

Salt and black pepper, to taste

4 medium butternut squash, peeled, seeded and sliced

3 tablespoons coconut cream

Pinch of nutmeg

2 tablespoons coconut oil

PREPARATIONS

1. Preheat the oven to 400 degrees F (200 degrees C).
2. Place chicken breasts in a bowl. Add red chilies, oregano, salt and black pepper and toss well.
3. Place chicken breasts in roasting pan.
4. Place butternut squash slices around chicken. Pour cream on butternut squash slices. Sprinkle with nutmeg, salt and black pepper.
5. Drizzle oil on chicken and butternut squash evenly.
6. Roast for 25 to 35 minutes.

NUTRITION FACTS PER SERVING

Calories: 446
Fat: 21.1g
Carbohydrates: 21.4g
Fiber: 5.9g
Sugar: 3.9g
Protein: 44.6g

Chicken with Coconut Milk

Prep Time: 10 minutes

Cooking Time: 1 hour 35 minutes

Serves: 4

Ingredients

1½ pound chicken thighs

Salt and black pepper, to taste

3 tablespoons coconut oil

2 cups coconut milk

10 cloves garlic, crushed

1 stick cinnamon

2 tablespoons fresh sage, chopped

Zest of 2 lemons, grated

PREPARATIONS

1. Preheat the oven to 375 degrees F (180 degrees C).
2. In a pan, heat oil on medium heat.
3. Add chicken and cook for 4 to 5 minutes.
4. Remove chicken from pan.
5. In a baking dish, add chicken and remaining ingredients and mix.
6. Bake for 1½ hours.

NUTRITION FACTS PER SERVING

Calories: 636
Fat: 44.1g
Carbohydrates: 10.2g
Fiber: 3.5g
Sugar: 4.1g
Protein: 52.6g

Mushrooms Stuffed Roasted Chicken

Prep Time: 10 minutes

Cooking Time: 1 hour 35 minutes

Serves: 4

Ingredients

4 tablespoons coconut oil, divided

4 cloves garlic, sliced finely

1 medium onion, chopped finely

1 pound mixed mushrooms, sliced

1 bunch fresh thyme, chopped

¼ cup pine nuts, chopped

1 large egg, beaten

2 pounds whole chicken

Zest of 1 lemon, grated

Salt and black pepper, to taste

Preparations

1. Preheat the oven to 475 degrees F (250 degrees C).
2. In a pan, heat 2 tablespoon of oil on medium heat.
3. Add garlic and onion and sauté for 8 to 10 minutes.
4. Add mushrooms and thyme and cook for 8 to 10 minutes.
5. Remove from heat and let it cool.
6. Stir in pine nuts and egg.
7. With your fingers, make a pocket between skin and meat.
8. Fill the pocket with ¼ of mushroom mixture.
9. Place half lemon zest in the cavity.
10. Place chicken in roasting pan and drizzle remaining oil. Season with salt and black pepper.
11. Roast for 40 minutes.
12. Place remaining mushroom stuffing in roasting tray and roast for 35 minutes more.

Nutrition Facts Per Serving

Calories: 546
Fat: 36.3g
Carbohydrates: 16.9g
Fiber: 4.2g
Sugar: 8.4g
Protein: 41.7g

Bacon with Apple & Avocado Salad

Prep Time: 15 minutes

Cooking Time: 15 minutes

Serves: 4

Ingredients

For Salad

¼ pound bacon, cut into ½-inch bits

8 boneless chicken thighs, cubed

¼ cup red onion, chopped

1 medium avocado, peeled, pitted and cubed

½ cup walnuts, chopped

1 green apple, cored and cubed

For Dressing

2 tablespoons apple cider

2 tablespoons lemon juice

1/3 cup extra-virgin olive oil

1 teaspoon Dijon mustard

2 cloves garlic, minced

Salt and black pepper, to taste

PREPARATIONS

1. In a nonstick pan, cook bacon on medium heat. Cook for 4 to 5 minutes or till crisp.
2. Remove bacon from pan.
3. In the same pan, add chicken. Season with salt and black pepper. Cook for 4 to 5 minutes or till browned.
4. Reduce heat to low. Simmer for 5 minutes more.
5. In a large bowl, add bacon, chicken, and remaining salad ingredients and mix.
6. In another bowl, add all dressing ingredients and whisk till well combined.
7. Pour dressing over salad and toss to coat well.

NUTRITION FACTS PER SERVING

Calories: 808
Fat: 57.8g
Carbohydrates: 17.1g
Fiber: 6.7g
Sugar: 8.0g
Protein: 60.2g

CRISPY CHICKEN WITH AVOCADO

Prep Time: 10 minutes

Cooking Time: 10 minutes

Serves: 4

INGREDIENTS

2 cups unsalted nuts (walnuts and almonds), chopped

2 cups fresh mixed herbs, chopped finely

Salt and black pepper, to taste

5 eggs

½ cup coconut oil

4 boneless chicken cutlets

3 avocadoes, peeled pitted and sliced

PREPARATIONS

1. In a bowl, mix together, nuts, herbs, salt and black pepper.
2. In another bowl, beat eggs.
3. In a frying pan, heat oil on medium heat.
4. Dip chicken cutlet in egg and then coat with nut and herb mixture.
5. Add chicken cutlet in pan and cook for 5 minutes per side or till browned.
6. Repeat with remaining cutlets.

NUTRITION FACTS PER SERVING

Calories: 941
Fat: 68.9g
Carbohydrates: 29.7g
Fiber: 20.3g
Sugar: 2.6g
Protein: 60.6g

Butter & Herbs Stuffed Chicken

Prep Time: 10 minutes

Cooking Time: 20 minutes

Serves: 4

Ingredients

½ cup almond butter, softened

1 tablespoon fresh parsley, chopped

1 tablespoon fresh dill, chopped

Salt and black pepper, to taste

4 (each 6-ounce) boneless chicken breasts

¼ cup coconut oil

1. In a bowl, add butter, herbs, salt and black pepper and mix till well combined.
2. Place butter in a plastic wrap and roll it into the shape of butter stick.
3. Place in freezer for 25 minutes.
4. With rolling pin, pound each chicken breast in ¼-inch thickness.
5. Divide butter into 4 equal portions.
6. Place a butter piece in the center of chicken. Roll the chicken tightly, so it covers the butter completely.
7. Refrigerate chicken for 1 to 2 hours.
8. In a pan, heat oil on medium-low heat.
9. Season the outer skin of chicken with salt and black pepper.
10. Cook chicken for 15 to 20 minutes or till browned from all sides.

NUTRITION FACTS PER SERVING

Calories: 641
Fat: 43.3g
Carbohydrates: 6g
Fiber: 1.3g
Sugar: 0.0g
Protein: 56g

STUFFED LAMB LEG WITH OLIVES

Prep Time: 10 minutes

Cooking Time: 1 hour

Serves: 4

INGREDIENTS

5 whole cloves garlic, peeled and divided

½ cup mixed fresh herbs (parsley, thyme, oregano)

½ cup almond meal

¼ cup pine nuts

½ cup green olives, pitted

Salt and black pepper to taste

2 pounds lamb leg

4 tablespoons coconut oil, divided

1 large bunch of rosemary

1 pound sweet potato, peeled and sliced

4 cups fresh lemon juice

1. Preheat the oven to 400 degrees F (200 degrees C).
2. In a food processor, add 3 cloves garlic and mixed herbs. Process till combined. Add almond meal and pulse for a while again.
3. Place the mixture in a bowl. Add some boiling water to form a thick paste.
4. Add in pine nuts and olives.
5. Place the stuffing in cavity of lamb. Brush with some oil and season with salt and pepper.
6. In a bowl add potatoes, remaining garlic, some oil, salt and black pepper and mix well.
7. Place lamb in the roasting tray.
8. Spread sweet potato slices around the lamb.
9. Roast for 1 hour.

NUTRITION FACTS PER SERVING

Calories: 297
Fat: 63.9g
Carbohydrates: 38.5g
Fiber: 11.3g
Sugar: 9.6g
Protein: 32.3g

LAMB SHANKS WITH RAISINS & HONEY

Prep Time: 10 minutes

Cooking Time: 3 hours 20 minutes

Serves: 4

INGREDIENTS

3 tablespoons coconut oil, divided

2 red onions

Salt and black pepper, to taste

3 tablespoons golden raisins

2 tablespoons tomato paste (home made)

1 tablespoon honey

4 lamb shanks (4-ounce each)

4 sprigs rosemary, chopped

2 cups chicken broth

2 scallions

1. In a pan, heat 1 tablespoon oil on medium-high heat.
2. Add onion and season with salt and black pepper. Sauté for 4 to 5 minutes.
3. Stir in raisins, honey, and tomato paste. Simmer for 5 minutes.
4. In another pan, heat remaining oil on medium-high heat.
5. Add lamb shanks and cook for 3 minutes per side.
6. Add rosemary and cook for 2 minutes.
7. Transfer lamb into the first pan with onions.
8. Add broth and bring to a boil. Reduce heat to medium-low. Cover and simmer for 3 hours.
9. Just before serving, stir in chopped scallions.

Nutrition Facts Per Serving

Calories: 288
Fat: 12.1g
Carbohydrates: 9.9g
Fiber: 0.9g
Sugar: 7.5g
Protein: 33.7g

CHICKEN & ORANGE SALAD

Prep Time: 10 minutes

Serves: 4

INGREDIENTS

4 cups cooked chicken, shredded

2 scallions, sliced finely

2 bunches lettuce, shredded

3 oranges, peeled, seeded and sectioned

3 tablespoons fresh lime juice

Salt and black pepper, to taste

1 cup walnuts

1. In a large salad bowl, add chicken, scallions, lettuce, and oranges. Drizzle lime juice and oil.
2. Season with salt and black pepper. Toss to coat well.

NUTRITION FACTS PER SERVING

Calories: 479
Fat: 22.9g
Carbohydrates: 21.7g
Fiber: 6.0g
Sugar: 14.2g
Protein: 49.8g

Chicken & Peas Soup

Prep Time: 10 minutes

Cooking Time: 45 minutes

Serves: 4

Ingredients

1 pound chicken, cut into bite size pieces

1 pound fresh peas, shelled

5 cups chicken broth

Salt, to taste

2 eggs, beaten

2 cups fresh spinach, chopped finely

1 teaspoon Coconut Vinegar

½ tablespoons lemon zest, grated

1. In a large soup pan, add chicken, peas, broth, and salt.
2. Bring to a boil on medium heat. Reduce the heat to low and simmer for about 30 to 40 minutes or till chicken and peas are done completely.
3. Now, add eggs slowly in soup, stirring continuously.
4. Stir in spinach, vinegar, and lemon zest. Season with salt and black pepper.

NUTRITION FACTS PER SERVING

Calories: 391
Fat: 12.8 g
Carbohydrates: 18.4g
Fiber: 6.2g
Sugar: 7.6g
Protein: 48.2g

Spicy Chicken with Lemongrass

Prep Time: 10 minutes

Cooking Time: 5 hours

Serves: 4

Ingredients

8 chicken drumsticks

Salt and black pepper, to taste

4 cloves garlic, minced

1 thick stalk fresh lemongrass trimmed and sliced

1 cup coconut milk

1 teaspoon ground cumin

1 teaspoon ground coriander

1 teaspoon all spice powder

1 large onion, sliced thinly

PREPARATIONS

1. In a bowl, add drumsticks and remaining ingredients except onion and mix well.
2. Spread onion slices in the bottom of slow cooker.
3. Place drumsticks with marinade on top.
4. Set the slow cooker on low. Cover and cook for 4 to 5 hours.

NUTRITION FACTS PER SERVING

Calories: 315

Fat: 19.7g

Carbohydrates: 7.9g

Fiber: 2.2g

Sugar: 3.5g

Protein: 27.3g

Curried Chicken with Bell Peppers

Prep Time: 10 minutes

Cooking Time: 4 hours

Serves: 4

Ingredients

1½ pounds boneless chicken thighs, cubed

1 small yellow onion, diced

½ head cabbage, shredded

1 green bell pepper, seeded and diced

1 red bell pepper, seeded and diced

2 cups coconut milk

3 tablespoons red curry paste

Salt and black pepper, to taste

PREPARATIONS

1. In a slow cooker, add all ingredients and mix well. Set the slow cooker on low.
2. Cover and cook for 4 hours.

NUTRITION FACTS PER SERVING

Calories: 692
Fat: 44.9g
Carbohydrates: 19.2g
Fiber: 6.5g
Sugar: 10.1g
Protein: 53.0g

Beef Steak with Vegetables

Prep Time: 10 minutes

Cooking Time: 8 hours 10 minutes

Serves: 4

Ingredients

3 tablespoons coconut oil, divided

1½ pounds beefsteak, cut into bite size pieces

1 small onion, chopped

2 stalks celery, chopped

2 medium carrots, peeled and chopped

1 tablespoon Italian seasoning

2 cups tomatoes, chopped

1 tablespoon coconut sugar

Salt and black pepper, to taste

2 cups fresh mushrooms, sliced

PREPARATIONS

1. In a pan, heat 2 tablespoons of oil on medium heat.
2. Add beef and cook for 10 minutes or till browned.
3. Transfer the beef into slow cooker.
4. In the same pan, add onion, celery, and carrots and sauté for 4 to 5 minutes.
5. Spread the mixture on beef in slow cooker and mix well.
6. Set the slow cooker on low. Cover and cook for 6 to 8 hours.
7. Meanwhile in a pan, heat remaining oil and sauté the mushrooms till brown.
8. Add the mushroom in slow cooker before 30 minutes of cooking is completed.

NUTRITION FACTS PER SERVING

Calories: 456
Fat: 22.1g
Carbohydrates: 9.2g
Fiber: 2.6g
Sugar: 5.2g
Protein: 53.9g

CHICKEN & SWEET POTATO SOUP

Prep Time: 10 minutes

Cooking Time: 40 minutes

Serves: 4

INGREDIENTS

3 tablespoons coconut oil

1 pound chicken, cut into bite size pieces

2 scallions, chopped

1 onion, chopped finely

2 teaspoons almond flour

4 cups chicken broth

½ pound sweet potatoes, diced finely

2 eggs, beaten

½ cup coconut cream

Salt and black pepper, to taste

3 teaspoons fresh parsley, chopped

1. In a soup pot, heat oil on medium-high heat.
2. Add chicken and cook for 5 minutes.
3. Transfer chicken into a plate.
4. In the same pan, add scallions and onions and cook for 4 to 5 minutes.
5. Stir in almond flour and cook for 1 minute.
6. Pour broth and sweet potatoes and bring to a boil.
7. Reduce heat to medium-low. Simmer for 15 to 20 minutes.
8. Add chicken and simmer for 10 minutes more.
9. In a bowl, add eggs, coconut cream and ½ cup soup and whisk well. Pour egg mixture in soup.
10. Simmer for 8 to 10 minutes

NUTRITION FACTS PER SERVING

Calories: 495
Fat: 21.4g
Carbohydrates: 30.4g
Fiber: 5.8g
Sugar: 5.5g
Protein: 46.0g

Roasted Chicken & Mashed Sweet Potatoes

Prep Time: 10 minutes

Cooking Time: 35 minutes

Serves: 4

Ingredients

1 pound boneless chicken fillets

2 teaspoons Dijon mustard

2 teaspoons honey

3 teaspoons fresh lemon juice

3 tablespoons coconut oil

Salt and black pepper, to taste

1 pound sweet potato, peeled and cubed

½ cup coconut milk

3 teaspoons fresh parsley, chopped finely

Preparations

1. Preheat the oven to 350 degrees F (175 degrees C). Line a baking pan with parchment paper
2. In a bowl, add mustard, honey lemon juice, ghee, salt and black pepper and mix well.
3. Add chicken and coat well.
4. Roast chicken fillet for 20-25 minutes or till chicken is done completely.
5. Meanwhile, steam the sweet potato chunks for 8 to 10 minutes.
6. Transfer the chunks to a bowl. Add coconut milk. Season with salt and black pepper.
7. Mash the chunks slightly.
8. Place chicken fillet and mashed sweet potatoes in a serving plate.
9. Garnish with chopped parsley.

Nutrition Facts Per Serving

Calories: 488
Fat: 26.1g
Carbohydrates: 28.3g
Fiber: 4.5g
Sugar: 11.3g
Protein: 36.0g

Beef Steak with Bell Peppers

Prep Time: 1 hour 10 minutes

Cooking Time: 35 minutes

Serves: 4

Ingredients

1 pound beef flank steaks

Salt and black pepper, to taste

1 teaspoon dried oregano

2 tablespoons coconut oil

1 onion, chopped

2 cloves garlic, chopped finely

1 cup beef broth

1 yellow bell pepper, diced

1 green bell pepper, diced

Fresh red jalapeno peppers

1. In a bowl combine beef, salt, black pepper, and oregano and mix well.
2. Cover and leave for 1 hour.
3. Heat oil in a pan; add in onion and cook for 3 minutes until browned.
4. Add garlic and cook for 2 minutes.
5. Add beef and cook for 5 minutes until tender. Stir in beef broth. Bring to a boil.
6. Cover and cook for 20 minutes on medium heat until beef is cooked and sauce is thickened.
7. Add in bell pepper, jalapeno peppers and cook for 5 minutes until softened.

NUTRITION FACTS PER SERVING

Calories: 311
Fat: 14.4g
Carbohydrates: 6.9g
Fiber: 2.0g
Sugar: 3.8g
Protein: 36.6g

Chicken & Avocado Soup

Prep Time: 10 minutes

Cooking Time: 40 minutes

Serves: 4

Ingredients

3 teaspoons coconut soup

2 garlic cloves, minced

1 tablespoon tomato paste (home made)

½ cup fresh tomatoes, chopped

½ avocado, thinly sliced

4 teaspoons chili powder

4 cups chicken broth

1 cup fresh beans, trimmed and chopped

Salt and black pepper, to taste

4 cups cooked chicken, shredded

¼ cup fresh cilantro leaves

1 scallion, thinly sliced

1. Heat oil in a pan on medium heat.
2. Add garlic and cook for 1 minute until fragrant.
3. Add tomato paste, tomatoes, avocado, and chili powder and cook 3 minutes until tomatoes are softened.
4. Add broth, beans, salt and pepper and bring to a boil. Reduce heat to medium-low.
5. Cover and cook for 30 minutes.
6. Add chicken, cilantro leaves, and scallion and cook for 5 minutes until cooked completely.

NUTRITION FACTS PER SERVING

Calories: 503
Fat: 13.9g
Carbohydrates: 37.1g
Fiber: 3.2g
Sugar: 3.2g
Protein: 57.3g

PAN FRIED CHICKEN

Prep Time: 10 minutes

Cooking Time: 15 minutes

Serves: 4

INGREDIENTS

4 tablespoons coconut oil

1 onion, sliced

5 garlic cloves, minced

1 pound chicken breast, strips

Salt and black pepper, to taste

2 green bell pepper, sliced

4 tomatoes, chopped

1 tablespoon diced green chilies

2 teaspoons chili powder

1 teaspoon cumin powder

¼ cup lemon juice

PREPARATIONS

1. Heat oil in a pan on medium heat.
2. Add onion and garlic and cook for 2 minutes until browned.
3. Add chicken, salt and pepper and cook for 8-10 minutes until tender.
4. Add in tomatoes, green chilies, green bell peppers, chili powder, and cumin and cook for 1 minute until softened.
5. Add in lemon juice and cook for 2 minutes until thickened.

NUTRITION FACTS PER SERVING

Calories: 372

Fat: 18.5g

Carbohydrates: 13.8g

Fiber: 4.1g

Sugar: 7.5g

Protein: 39.1g

CURRIED SHRIMP

Prep Time: 10 minutes

Cooking Time: 15 minutes

Serves: 4

INGREDIENTS

1 pound large shrimps, peeled

4 tablespoons coconut oil

1 onion, chopped

2 teaspoons fresh ginger, minced

4 cloves garlic

½ cup tomatoes, pureed

½ teaspoon ground cumin

½ teaspoon ground coriander

½ teaspoon turmeric

3 tablespoons fresh lime juice

PREPARATIONS

1. Heat oil in a pan on medium heat.
2. Add onion, ginger and garlic and cook for 5 minutes until tender.
3. Add shrimps and cook for 7-8 minutes until softened.
4. Add tomatoes, cumin, coriander, and turmeric and cook for 2 minutes.
5. Add in lime juice.

NUTRITION FACTS PER SERVING

Calories: 235
Fat: 13.8g
Carbohydrates: 8.1g
Fiber: 1.1g
Sugar: 1.9g
Protein: 22.1g

Fish Stew

Prep Time: 10 minutes

Cooking Time: 30 minutes

Serves: 4

Ingredients

2 tablespoons coconut oil

3 tomatoes, chopped

¼ pound bacon bits

¼ pound cabbage, sliced

½ pound sweet potatoes, cubed

Salt and black pepper, to taste

1 pound Salmon Fillets

2 tablespoons fresh lemon juice

6 cups fish broth

1 tablespoon chopped cilantro

1. Heat oil in a pan on medium heat.
2. Add tomatoes, bacon and cabbage and cook for 5 minutes.
3. Now add in sweet potatoes, salt and pepper and cook for 5 minutes or till tender.
4. Add fish and lemon juice and cook for 8 to10 minutes or till tender.
5. Add broth. Bring to a boil. Cover and cook for 15 minutes or till fish cooks completely.
6. Top with cilantro.

Nutrition Facts Per Serving

Calories: 535
Fat: 27.4g
Carbohydrates: 24.8g
Fiber: 5.8g
Sugar: 5.3g
Protein: 43.1g

Baked Fish Fillets

Prep Time: 10 minutes

Cooking Time: 30 minutes

Serves: 4

Ingredients

1 pound salmon fillets

2 cups almond flour

1 cup coconut flour

Salt and black pepper, to taste

4 eggs, beaten

4 tablespoons almond butter, melted

PREPARATIONS

1. Preheat the oven to 450 degrees F/225 degrees C. Grease a baking dish.
2. In a bowl, mix together almond flour, coconut flour, salt and black pepper.
3. In another bowl, whisk together eggs
4. Dip the fish in the beaten eggs first. Then coat with the flour mixture.
5. Place fish fillets in prepared baking dish. Brush fish fillets with melted butter.
6. Bake for 20 to 30 minutes or till golden brown.

NUTRITION FACTS PER SERVING

Calories: 439
Fat: 23.49
Carbohydrates: 18.3g
Fiber: 10.9g
Sugar: 2.3g
Protein: 32.8g

STIR FRY SHRIMPS & VEGETABLES

Prep Time: 10 minutes

Cooking Time: 25 minutes

Serves: 4

INGREDIENTS

3 tablespoons coconut oil, divided

1½ pounds shrimp

1 onion, sliced

5 cloves garlic, chopped

2 carrots, sliced

2 tablespoons water chestnuts, sliced

4 cups cabbage, shredded

Salt and black pepper, to taste

2 tablespoons fresh lime juice

PREPARATIONS

1. Heat 1 tablespoon oil in a pan on medium heat.
2. Add shrimps and cook for 10 minutes or till tender. Remove from pan and keep aside.
3. Heat remaining oil in the pan.
4. Add onion and garlic and cook for 2 minutes or till softened.
5. Now add in carrot, water chestnuts, cabbage and cook for 3 minutes until tender.
6. Add shrimps salt and juice and cook for 5 minutes.

NUTRITION FACTS PER SERVING

Calories: 334
Fat: 13.3g
Carbohydrates: 18.8g
Fiber: 3.3
Sugars: 5.0g
Protein: 40.8g

CREAMY CHICKEN WITH MUSTARD

Prep Time: 10 minutes

Cooking Time: 20 minutes

Serves: 4

INGREDIENTS

4 chicken boneless breasts

Salt and black pepper, to taste

3 tablespoons coconut oil

1 onion, chopped finely

4 cloves garlic, chopped finely

3 teaspoons almond flour

1 tablespoon Dijon mustard

2 cups chicken broth

4 tablespoon tarragon, divided

2 tablespoons coconut cream

1. Preheat the oven to 375 degrees F/180 degrees C. Lightly, grease a baking dish.
2. Season chicken with salt and black pepper.
3. In a pan, heat oil on medium heat.
4. Add chicken and cook for 2 to 3 minutes per side or till golden. Remove from pan and keep aside.
5. Add onion and garlic and sauté for 2-3 minutes.
6. Add almond flour and cook, stirring for about 30 seconds.
7. Add mustard, broth and tarragon and bring to a boil, stirring continuously.
8. Add chicken in the pan.
9. Transfer the chicken mixture into a baking dish.
10. Bake for 8 to 10 minutes or till chicken is done completely.
11. Transfer the mixture again to pan. Remove chicken from pan. Place pan on medium-high heat and cook for 2 to 3 minutes or till sauce thickens.
12. Stir in cream and heat completely.
13. Place chicken in plate. Pour sauce over chicken.
14. Top with tarragon leaves and serve.

NUTRITION FACTS PER SERVING

Calories: 529
Fat: 33.7g
Carbohydrates: 9.1g
Fiber: 3.2g
Sugars: 2.5g
Protein: 48.2g

Chicken & Tomatoes

Prep Time: 10 minutes

Cooking Time: 1 hour 30 minutes

Serves: 4

Ingredients

8 chicken drumsticks

Salt and black pepper, to taste

1 bunch basil, chopped

1½ cups cherry tomatoes, halved

1½ cups plum tomatoes, quartered

5 cloves garlic

2 fresh red chilies, seeded and sliced

3 tablespoons coconut butter, melted

PREPARATIONS

1. Preheat the oven to 350 degrees F (175 degrees C).
2. Season chicken with salt and black pepper.
3. Spread basil, tomatoes and garlic cloves in the baking dish.
4. Place chicken in the center of baking dish.
5. Bake for 1½ hours.
6. Remove garlic before serving

NUTRITION FACTS PER SERVING

Calories: 400
Fat: 21.8g
Carbohydrates: 23.3g
Fiber: 8.5g
Sugars: 13.1g
Protein: 30.7g

CRISPY CHICKEN WITH ASPARAGUS & TOMATOES

Prep Time: 10 minutes

Cooking Time: 15 minutes

Serves: 4

INGREDIENTS

4 chicken breasts, cut into strips

Salt and black pepper, to taste

3 tablespoons coconut oil

2 bunches asparagus, trimmed

½ pound cherry tomatoes, halved

10 black olives, pitted

½ cup fresh basil, chopped

2 tablespoons coconut butter

¼ cup chicken broth

PREPARATIONS

1. Season chicken with salt and black pepper.
2. In a large skillet, heat oil on medium heat.
3. Add chicken and asparagus and cook, stirring often for 10 minutes.
4. With a spoon, move chicken and asparagus to one side of skillet.
5. Add olives, tomatoes, basil and butter in skillet.
6. Add chicken broth.
7. Cook for 4 to 5 minutes or till thickens.

NUTRITION FACTS PER SERVING

Calories: 304
Fat: 14.5g
Carbohydrates: 8.1g
Fiber: 3.6g
Sugars: 4.5g
Protein: 35.7g

CRISPY CHICKEN WITH GREEN CURRY & SLAW

Prep Time: 15 minutes

Cooking Time: 30 minutes

Serves: 4

INGREDIENTS

For Slaw

1 red onion, sliced thinly

1 small bunch radishes, sliced thinly

½ head cabbage, shredded

1 red chili, seeded and sliced

1 green chili, seeded and sliced

1 bunch fresh coriander

For Chicken

2 tablespoons coconut milk

1½ pounds chicken thighs

2 tablespoons sesame seeds

Salt and black pepper, to taste

2 tablespoons honey

For Green Curry Sauce

2 tablespoons coconut oil

1 (2-inch) piece fresh ginger

2 fresh red chilies, seeded and sliced

4 kaffir lime leaves

4 cloves garlic

1 stick lemongrass

1 bunch scallions, sliced

1 bunch fresh coriander

1 ½ cup chicken broth

1 cup fresh beans, trimmed

1 ½ cups coconut milk

2 limes, juiced

PREPARATIONS

1. In a bowl, add onion, radishes, and cabbage.
2. In a blender, add red and green chili and coriander and pulse till smooth. Add into vegetables and mix. Refrigerate to chill.
3. In a pan, heat oil on medium heat.
4. Add chicken and season with salt and black pepper.
5. Cook, turning often for 18 to 20 minutes.

6. Meanwhile, in a blender, add oil, ginger, red chilies, lime leaves, garlic, lemongrass, scallions, and coriander. Blend till smooth.
7. Remove fats from chicken. Stir in 2 tablespoons of curry paste in chicken. Add sesame seeds and honey and toss well.
8. Heat another pan on medium heat.
9. Add remaining curry paste, broth, and coconut milk. Bring to a boil.
10. Reduce the heat to low. Add lime juice and cook till the sauce thickens.
11. Serve chicken with green sauce and slaw.

NUTRITION FACTS PER SERVING

Calories: 735
Fat: 45.6g
Carbohydrates: 29.6g
Fiber: 7.4g
Sugar: 17.1g
Protein: 56.4g

WHY ARE SO MANY PEOPLE FAILING? GET MY FREE REPORT

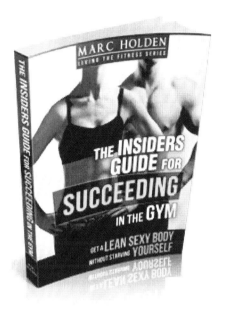

A lot of people seem to be failing after all the hard work in the gym. There is #1 reason why these people (and maybe you?) are failing and wasting their time in the gym right now.

In this free report I explain how you can succeed in your home gym. So grab your free copy of '**The Insiders Guide for Succeeding in the Gym**' now at livingthefitness.com/succeeding-gym/ and get that body you desire.

Thank You!

Thanks a lot for reading my book. If you like this book, please leave me a good review on Amazon. It's the best compliment I can get and it will help more people to find my book easily.

Become a fan on Facebook for free content. Join us today at **facebook.com/livingthefitness**. I share here great articles about fitness and nutrition.

When you're interested in more books of the Living the Fitness series, please sign up for my free newsletter at **www.livingthefitness.com**.

Free Book Excerpt

Are you bored with your workouts? Looking for something new? Something better?

CrossFit infuses team spirit and good-natured competition in fitness.

CrossFit for Beginner makes getting in shape and staying that way fun!

Want to discover what you were missing all those years? Grab your copy of my book at **Amazon.com**.

Excerpt from 'CrossFit for Beginners: Get Muscle, Strenth and Stamina in 30 Minutes or Less'

CROSSFIT TRAINING

CrossFit targets ten domains of fitness. These domains include cardiovascular and respiratory endurance, stamina, strength, flexibility, power, speed, coordination, balance, agility and accuracy. The entire philosophy of CrossFit training is that all ten of these areas must be trained in order to achieve true fitness. CrossFit is purposefully designed to be intense, physically demanding, and enervating. Because of this, it is optimal training for the military and athletes. But if you are not part of these groups, never fear. CrossFit is highly adaptable and can be adjusted to work with anybody and any skill level. Generally, it is recommended that you work with an affiliated gym for with a certified trainer, especially if you are a beginner fitness athlete. So, what does CrossFit training look like?

LIFTING WEIGHTS

CrossFit uses weights. And if you are looking at the CrossFit website for WOD or other games, you may notice that the prescribed weight is much more than you can lift. CrossFit targets CrossFit men, generally. But you can adapt the weight to meet your needs. You can use lighter barbells or even just a PVC pipe if you have to. Especially in the beginning stages, CrossFit training is very concerned with form; that is, how you lift a weight. CrossFit will ask that you maintain certain positions while lifting weights, and not try to work around form just to lift a weight (badly) once or twice. CrossFit's entire goal is to get you fit enough to lift weights with good form and range of motion. More important is the number of repetitions that you can complete using the correct form. So if the WOD asks for lifting 50 pounds over your head 25 times, then adjust as needed. But keep the 25 reps. Maybe lift 10 pounds 25 times with excellent form.

RESISTANCE TRAINING

CrossFit loves to use your own body weight as resistance for things like pull ups, squats, pushups and handstand pushups. For most people, these training exercises will have to be adapted. So, if you cannot do a handstand push up, then you can, instead, do pushups on an inclined plane by putting your feet on a box that is one foot off the ground. Again, what is important is form. So be sure to do form-perfect exercises, even if you cannot do the prescribed level of resistance.

To look at another example, suppose the WOD asks you to do squat while resting 250 LBS on your back shoulders. CrossFit considers the squat a basic movement and is prevalent in many training routines. Ok. For most of us, this is not possible today. So, instead, focus on doing the toughest squat you can. This may mean that you squat with no weights and a bar for support, but do 50. Or it may mean that you squat with 20 pounds across your shoulders, with no bar for support 5 times. Focus on form and range of motion and balance. These are the key elements to the CrossFit philosophy.

ENDURANCE

CrossFit never said that their routines were comfortable. You will be pushed to your limit and endurance training is one of the ways CrossFit does this. High intensity for CrossFit means high average. So, if a beginner fitness athlete can maintain 3.2 MPH on a treadmill for 30 minutes, a high averaged one would be able to maintain about a 4.2 MPH pace just to give you an idea. So, CrossFit wants you to push yourself to your limits, but not so much that you get sick or injure yourself. What is more important is that you are able to maintain the given activity for the length of time set (usually 20 minutes). You should be able to breathe even though you are pushing yourself to maintain a constant flow of motion.

Remember that for CrossFit, this is a sport: "the sport of fitness". So, like any sport, it is necessary to keep track of what you were able to accomplish during a training workout. CrossFit has two ways to measure progress; time and number of repetitions. There are many ways to record your progress. You can use "old school" ways like a journal or index cards. Or you can use iPhone apps and other online tools to record your WODs. Whatever method you use, be sure that you state any weight you used, or modification, and how long you were able to maintain the activity. So, if you did 30 squats, but needed the support of a bar, be sure to document this. One day, you will do 30 squats without any support. You will want to know how long it took you to be able to do this task.

End excerpt from 'CrossFit for Beginners: Get Muscle, Strenth and Stamina in 30 Minutes or Less'

If you are interested in getting the body of your dreams and start learning more about CrossFit, go ahead and grab your copy today at **Amazon.com**!

Take care,

Marc

Living the fitness

Medical Disclaimer

The information in this book is for educational purposes only. It is not meant to provide or replace medical advice you may have received. If you are concerned about a medical or health issue, contact your health care provider immediately. If you are pregnant, have a major health issue, are under 18 or over 65, do not embark on any dietary changes without consulting your physician or other health care provider.

The dietary suggestions in this book are not meant to cure an illness. Your first line of defense in promoting good health is always a consultation with your health care provider. Feel free to discuss this book with your doctor or nutritionist and tailor the book and recipes to your own needs.

Printed in Great Britain
by Amazon